THE COMPLETE
KETO DIET GUIDE
TO LOSE WEIGHT

Delicious and Affordable Keto Recipes for Beginners and Pros
incl. 14 Days Weight Loss Plan

Emma Louise Bailey

Copyright © [2019] [Emma Louise Bailey]

All rights reserved

The author of this book owns the exclusive right to its content.
Any commercial usage or reproduction requires the clear consent of the author.

ISBN- 9798629496366

TABLE OF CONTENTS

Keto Diet: Things You Need to Know 6
How the Body Changes during the Keto Diet 7
How to Lose Weight Effectively on the Keto Diet 8
How to Lose up to 20 Pounds in 3 Weeks 9
Recipes 11
Breakfast (15 recipes) 12
    Almond Flour Bread 13
    Egg Rollups 14
    Sausage Casserole 15
    Vegan Porridge 16
    Bulletproof Coffee 17
    Ham & Cheese Pockets 18
    French Toast from Scratch 19
    Salted Caramel Pork Rind Cereal 20
    Chia Pudding 21
    Spinach & Sausage Muffin 22
    Strawberry Smoothie 23
    Crunchy Energy Bars 24
    Mocha Mousse 25
    Egg Burrito 26
    Cheesy Breakfast Bowl 27
Lunch (15 recipes) 28
    Fried Cauliflower and Cheese Patties 29
    Creamed Spinach 30
    Indian Style Chicken Curry 31
    Salmon Patties with Tartar Sauce 33

TABLE OF CONTENTS

- Bacon & Cheeseburger Soup 35
- Cheesy Lettuce Wraps 36
- No-Cook Lunch Box 37
- Cobb Salad 38
- Oven-baked Chicken Parmesan 39
- Stuffed Tomatoes 41
- Zucchini Bolognese 42
- Steamed Pork Cabbage Rolls 44
- Avocado & Egg Salad Bowl 46
- Lunchbox Omelette 47
- Classic Caprese 48

Dinner (15 Recipes) 49
- Mashed Cauliflower 50
- Chicken & Mushroom Stew 51
- Buffalo Chicken Soup 52
- Crunchy Bread Rolls 53
- Eggplant Parmesan 54
- Tuna Salad 55
- Pork Chops with Caramelized Onion 56
- Oven-Baked Meatloaf 57
- Chicken & Green Beans Almondine 58
- Salisbury Steak in Slow Cooker 60
- Mexican Style Cauliflower Rice 62
- Shrimp Alfredo 64
- Thai Spicy Tofu 66
- Asian Style Stir-Fried Veggies 67

TABLE OF CONTENTS

    Creamy Garlic Mushrooms 68
Snacks & Desserts (8 Recipes) 70
    Pepperoni Pizza 71
    Flourless Brownies 73
    Keto Microwave Mug Cake 75
    Pizza Chips 76
    Cheesy Breadsticks 77
    Coconut Cashew Bars 78
    Sauteed Mushrooms 79
    Tortilla Chips 80
14 Days Weight Loss and Meal Plan (how to lose up to 11 pounds in 14 days) 81

[Handwritten notes:]

1 lb (pound) = 454 g

1 oz (ounce) = 28.3 g

'Keto Diet' or 'Ketogenic Diet' is one of the widely followed diet methods that helps one to improve his health in numerous ways. In contrast to most diets, ketogenic diet focuses more on high-fat food items and does not encourage limiting food intake. One can benefit from this diet by lessening the amount of carbohydrate or starch-based foods. An average keto diet consists of about 85% healthy fats, 20% protein and 5% carbs. Depending on the body type and the health condition, one can alter the ratio and maintain the diet suitable for his body type.

Keto diet works well with almost everyone because of its massive impact on the body previously used to carbs. With an added emphasis on the fats, the body is forced to go into a different metabolic state known as ketosis. In this process, the fat turns into ketones which transforms into energy that reaches the brain. This is why the body fat is burned faster than usual. The process is especially beneficial to the obese or over-weight people who may notice a major change in their body fat after following the keto diet. Keto also lowers the insulin and blood sugar levels, thus making the body more fit and energetic over time.

When one starts following the keto diet, the body changes rapidly. Depending on the body type, it may take 24-72 hours to get into the ketogenic state. Many people try intermittent fasting for 24 hours to get into ketogenic state faster. Once the body gets in this state, one may notice numerous changes in the body, both positive and negative. Here are some of the most common changes that may appear when you are following a keto diet:

Rapid Weight Loss
Maintaining a balanced calorie diet with the right amount of fat, protein and carb intake can cause faster weight loss. Combined with exercise, keto diet may help one to lose up to 20 pounds in 3 weeks.

Reaction to Carb Withdrawal
Widely known as the 'keto flu', different physical reactions to keto diet may occur if someone is new to keto diet. Insomnia, headache, fatigue, mood swings, etc. are common in the first 2-3 days of keto diet. Many people also suffer from constipation, bowel problems, rashes, etc. right after starting keto. However, this passes once the induction phase is over and the body gains more energy than before.

Improved Insulin Sensitivity
Without carbohydrate and sugar, the blood sugar levels lessen. This is especially beneficial for the people suffering from type 2 diabetes, as it helps to increase insulin sensitivity.

Increased Energy Level
Once the body is adapted to the keto diet, the energy levels start to stabilize and increase in many cases. The brain is fully charged and stimulates various physical and psychological functions to perform better than before.

Reduced Inflammation and Skin Diseases
Inflammation is one of the major causes that leads to heart diseases, bowel diseases and cancer. Maintaining a keto diet may lower the inflammation in the body. It may also improve eczema, arthritis, Crohn's disease, hormonal acne and many other health conditions caused by unhealthy eating habits.

Many studies show that one can actually reduce weight and improve health condition by maintaining the keto diet. In fact, people may lose weight 2.2 times faster than the people who maintain diets that restrict calories or food intake.

The secret of the success of keto diet lies mostly in its perfect balance of protein and fat intake. While the fat is burned to produce energy, protein and leafy greens help one to keep the body packed with necessary nutrients. Unlike other diets, daily average calorie count of 2000 kcal is maintained in keto diet. This is another reason why keto followers can enjoy wholesome meals throughout the day and gain faster results at the same time.

In order to lose weight with the keto diet, one needs to avoid certain food items. Starchy foods like cereal, rice, pasta, noodles, etc. must be avoided. Sugary foods, root vegetables, unhealthy and artificial fats, majority of the fruits should also be restricted in a keto diet.

To fill the body with the beneficial nutrients and boost up weight loss, certain foods must be added to the diet. Butter, olive oil, coconut oil, cheese, nuts, herbs and spices, meat, fish and leafy greens, mushrooms, seafood etc. work excellent in this case. With the right foods added to the daily meals, losing weight can be fast and effortless over time.

While losing weight on keto diet may seem faster than any other diet methods, the progress of weight loss may not work the same for everyone. However, it is possible to achieve the best outcome by following a few strategies. Here's how they work:

Avoid Carb and Sugar
As almost every food item has some percentage of carbohydrates in it, it is almost impossible to avoid carb completely. To balance the daily carb intake, avoid foods with whole carbs (rice, pasta, noodles, etc.) Swap for foods like cauliflower, eggplant, cucumber and cherry tomatoes that are low on carb.

As for the sugary foods, avoid honey, white sugar, brown sugar, etc. and try to use coconut milk, coconut cream, Stevia or similar artificial sweeteners while preparing a sugary dessert.

Create a Meal Plan
Creating a meal plan beforehand will help you to prepare dish easily and make keto diet simpler. It will also help you to decide on your weekly shopping and count your daily intakes.

Swap for Healthier Food Versions
Almost all regular food items can be tried out using keto-approved food ingredients. You can use coconut flour, almond flour, psyllium husk, flaxseed meal, hemp seeds in flour-based recipes. Regular oil can be swapped for coconut oil or olive oil. You can substitute milk for coconut milk or almond milk. Pasta or noodles can also be tried out with zucchini or cucumber. Similarly, cauliflower rice can be used as an alternative of regular rice. Opt for healthy recipes to make keto diet a manageable lifestyle instead of a strict diet.

Squeeze in a Snack Time
Apart from 3 meals a day, it is also important to add snack time in your diet plan. It will keep your unhealthy cravings on check and help you to continue with the diet without feeling starved. Munch on nuts, roasted seeds, homemade granola bars or keto-friendly snack items. You can also make keto icecream, keto fat bombs or chocolate desserts and store in the refrigerator for later.

Save Some Time for Exercise

Regular exercise during the keto diet helps one to lose weight a lot faster than those who rely on the diet only. If you cannot find time to attend gym, try to do free-hand exercises at home. This will burn all the extra calories and tone your body faster than ever.

RECIPES

If you are planning on starting a keto diet, check out the following recipes for inspiration:

BREAKFAST (15 RECIPES)

1

Time: 5 minutes| Servings: 4
Serving: 1 slice
Net Carbs: 1g / 0.03oz
Fat: 7.5g / 0.26oz
Protein: 6g / 0.21oz
Fiber: 1.5g / 0.05oz
Kcal: 104

INGREDIENTS:

- ½ cup Almond Flour (blanched)
- ½ tsp. Confectioners Erythritol
- ½ tsp. Baking Powder
- ½ scoop Whey Protein (Unflavoured)
- ¼ tsp. Xanthan Gum
- 2.5 oz Water

INSTRUCTIONS:

1. Mix all the ingredients in a mixing bowl and form a thick batter.
2. Coat a small Tupperware baking dish with baking spray and pour the batter into it. Make sure that the batter is evenly spread.
3. Microwave for 1-2 minutes depending on the temperature of your oven.
4. Let the bread cool down.
5. Slice into 4 pieces and serve with your favourite keto spread on top.

ALMOND FLOUR BREAD

EGG ROLLUPS

2

Time: 25 minutes | Servings: 5
Serving: 1
Net carbs: 2.26g / 0.07oz
Fat: 31.66g / 1.12oz
Protein: 28.21g / 0.99oz
kcal: 412.2

INGREDIENTS:

- 10 large Eggs
- 1.5 cups shredded Cheddar Cheese
- 5 slices cooked Bacon
- 5 patties cooked Sausage
- Nonstick Cooking Spray
- Pinch of Salt
- Pinch of Pepper

INSTRUCTIONS:

1. Heat up a nonstick skillet. Keep the heat medium-high and spray on some nonstick cooking spray.

2. Whisk 2 eggs in a mixing bowl. Pour the mixture in the skillet and turn the heat medium-low. Sprinkle some salt and pepper.

3. Cover with a lid for a few minutes, until the egg is half cooked. Sprinkle some cheese and place a slice of bacon and one sausage patty on top.

4. Roll the egg from the sides to the middle so that it covers the fillings.

5. Flip over the egg to cook both the sides. Remove from the pan when it's done.

6. Repeat the process 4 more times until you have 5 rollups. Serve warm.

3

Time: 15 minutes | Servings: 4
Serving: 1
Net carbs: 3.86g / 0.14oz
Fat: 39.76g / 1.40oz
Protein: 22.08g / 0.78oz
kcal: 468.3

INGREDIENTS:

- 1 pound Pork Sausage
- 2 cups Cabbage (Shredded)
- 2 cups Zucchini (Diced)
- 3 large eggs
- ½ cup Onion (Diced)
- ½ cup Mayonnaise
- 1 ½ cups Cheddar Cheese (Shredded)
- 2 tsp. Yellow Mustard
- 1 tsp. Sage (Dried and Ground)
- Pinch of Cayenne Pepper

INSTRUCTIONS:

1. Preheat the oven to 375°F. Grease a medium-sized casserole dish and set aside.
2. Cook the sausage halfway through in a large skillet. Keep the heat medium.
3. Add shredded cabbage, onion and zucchini. Remove from the skillet when the veggies are tender and the sausage is cooked all the way through.
4. Place the mixture into the casserole dish and set aside.
5. Whisk the eggs with sage, mayonnaise, mustard and pepper until a smooth consistency forms. Add 1 cup of cheese in the mixture and stir a few times.
6. Pour the egg mixture over the sausage and veggies in the casserole dish. Top with the remaining ½ cup of cheese.
7. Place casserole in the oven and bake for 30 minutes until the cheese is lightly browned on top.

SAUSAGE CASSEROLE

VEGAN PORRIDGE

4

Time: 15 minutes | Serves 2
Serving: 1
Net carbs: 5.78g / 0.20oz
Fat: 13.07g / 0.46oz
Protein: 17.82g / 0.63oz
Kcal: 249

INGREDIENTS:

- 2 tbsp. Coconut Flour
- 3 tbsp. golden Flaxseed Meal
- 1 ½ cups Almond Milk
- 2 tbsp vegan Vanilla Protein Powder
- Powdered Erythritol

INSTRUCTIONS:

1. Mix all the dry ingredients together in a bowl.
2. Put the mixture in a saucepan. Pour the almond milk and combine everything together. Stir every once in a while to ensure nothing sticks to the pan.
3. Add the sweetener according to your preference when the mixture thickens up.
4. Pour the porridge on a bowl and serve with your favorite toppings.

5

Time: 10 minutes | Serving: 1
Serving: 1
Net Carbs: 1g / 0.03oz
Fat: 29g / 1.09oz
Kcal: 268

INGREDIENTS:

- 12 oz brewed Coffee
- 2 tbsp. Ghee
- 1 tbsp. MCT oil
- 1/4 tsp. Pink Salt (Optional)
- Stevia (To Taste)
- 1/2 tsp. Cinnamon Powder

INSTRUCTIONS:

1. Brew 12 ounce of coffee using your preferred brewing method.
2. Pour all the ingredients in a blender and blend until a smooth consistency forms.
3. Serve hot or cold by adding ice cubes.
4. Add protein powder, cocoa powder or other ingredients to alter the taste each time you try this recipe.

HAM & CHEESE POCKETS

6

Time: 30 minutes | Servings: 2
Serving: 1
Net carbs: 4.2g / 0.15oz
Fat: 31g / 1.09oz
Protein: 31.7g / 1.12oz
Kcal: 426

INGREDIENTS:

- 3 oz Mozzarella Cheese (Shredded)
- 3 oz Ham
- 3 oz Cheddar Cheese
- 1 tbsp Cream Cheese
- 4 tbsp Flax Meal

INSTRUCTIONS:

1. Melt the shredded mozzarella and the cream cheese in the microwave and add in the flax meal. Mix everything together.
2. When the dough is formed, roll it thinly between two parchment paper sheets.
3. Put slices of ham in the middle and top with cheddar cheese slices.
4. Fold the dough over the filling from all four sides, like an envelope. Poke a few holes here and there for releasing steam during the cooking process.
5. Bake for 15-20 minutes on 400°F. Remove from the oven when the dough turns golden brown.
6. Let it cool down for a minute or two. Eat while it's hot to experience the melted cheesy texture.

7

Time: 60 minutes | Servings: 8
Net carbs: 2.5g / 0.09oz
Fat: 20.6g / 0.73oz
Protein: 5.7g / 0.20oz
Kcal: 232

INGREDIENTS:

- 8 oz Cream Cheese
- 4 medium-sized Eggs
- ¼ cup Coconut Flour
- 4 tbsp melted Butter
- ¼ cup Heavy Cream
- 1 tsp Vanilla Essence
- 2 tsp Baking Powder
- 1 tsp Cinnamon Powder
- Stevia to taste

INSTRUCTIONS:

1. Preheat the oven to 350°F.
2. Add all the ingredients in a blender. Pulse a few times until the cheese is fully blended with the remaining ingredients.
3. Damp a parchment paper. Line a loaf pan with the damp parchment paper. Make sure to leave an extra inch of paper on the sides for pulling out the loaf later.
4. Bake the loaf at for 45 minutes at 350°F. Slice the loaf when it cools down.
5. Heat up 1-2 tbsp of butter on an a skillet. Put one slice and cook until both sides are crisp and golden brown. Serve with maple syrup on top. You can also add fresh berries or banana slices to satisfy your cravings.

FRENCH TOAST FROM SCRATCH

SALTED CARAMEL PORK RIND CEREAL

8

Time: 60 minutes | Servings: 1
Serving: 1 bowl
Net carbs: 2.05g / 0.07oz
Fat: 48.38g / 1.71oz
Protein: 17.12g / 0.60oz
Kcal: 514

INGREDIENTS:

- 1 oz Pork Rinds
- 1 cup Coconut Milk
- 2 tbsp Heavy Whipping Cream
- 2 tbsp melted Butter
- 1 tbsp Erythritol
- ½ tsp Vanilla Essence
- ¼ tsp ground Cinnamon

INSTRUCTIONS:

1. Break the pork rinds into your preferred cereal size pieces.
2. Heat up the butter over medium heat. Remove from the heat when it starts to brown up.
3. Add heavy cream and erythritol into the butter and mix everything together.
4. Turn on the heat to a medium and let the mixture turn into a caramel.
5. Add the pork rinds into the caramel. Make sure all the rinds are evenly coated.
6. Remove from the pan and put the pork rinds in a container.
7. Let it cool in the refrigerator for 30-45 minutes.
8. Serve in a small bowl with almond milk and other favourite toppings.

9

Time: 6-8 hours | Servings: 1
Serving: 1 bowl
Net carbs: 12.5g / 0.44oz
Fiber: 11g / 0.38oz
Fat: 10g / 0.35oz
Protein: 5g / 0.18oz
Kcal: 151

INGREDIENTS:

- 2 tbsp. of Chia Seeds
- 2/3 drops of liquid Stevia
- 1 cup Coconut Milk
- Fresh Berries
- Chopped Nuts

INSTRUCTIONS:

1. In a small bowl, add the chia seeds and the coconut milk. Leave it in the refrigerator for 6-8 hours.
2. Mix stevia or any healthy sweetener according to your taste. Top with nuts and fresh berries for a hearty breakfast.

CHIA PUDDING

SAVOURY BREAKFAST MUFFIN

10

Time: 35 minutes | Servings: 9
Serving: 1 cup
Net carbs: 3.22g / 0.11oz
Fiber: 4g / 0.14oz
Fat: 28.7g / 1.01oz
Protein: 8.6g / 0.30oz
Kcal: 319

INGREDIENTS:

- 1 cup Macadamia Nuts (Roasted)
- ¾ cup Coconut Butter
- 5 medium-sized Eggs
- 1 tsp Baking Soda
- ½ tspn Kosher Salt
- ½ tsp Lemon Zest
- 1 tbsp Lemon Juice
- 1 cup Feta Cheese
- 1 cup Spinach
- 3 tbsp Parmesan Cheese (Grated)

INSTRUCTIONS:

1. Preheat the oven to 350°F.
2. Put the macadamia nuts in a food processor and blend into a creamy texture.
3. During the process, add the eggs one at a time.
4. Turn off the machine and put the coconut butter and salt. Combine these with the egg mixture and blend again. Lastly, add baking soda, lemon juice and lemon zest. Blend for another 10 seconds.
5. Put the batter on a large bowl. Add the spinach and the feta cheese. Mix well.
6. Rub butter on a muffin tin. Fill the tins halfway through and top with bits of grated parmesan cheese.
7. Bake for 25 minutes until the top turns golden brown.
8. Serve when it cools down a bit.

11

Time: 5 minutes | Servings: 1
Serving: 1 Glass
Net carbs: 7g / 0.24oz
Fiber: 3g / 0.10oz
Fat: 10g / 0.35oz
Protein: 23g / 0.81oz
Kcal: 215

INGREDIENTS:

- 1 cup Almond Milk
- 1/4 cup of Frozen Strawberries
- 1 tbsp Greek Yoghurt
- 1 tsp vanilla extract
- 30g Protein Powder
- 1/5 tsp Coconut Oil
- Pinch of Salt

INSTRUCTIONS:

1. Chop up the frozen strawberries for faster processing.
2. Put all the ingredients in a blender and pulse for 1/1.5 minutes. You will be looking for a thick, smooth texture.
3. Pour it into a glass.
4. Top with chopped strawberries or crushed nuts.

STRAWBERRY SMOOTHIE

CRUNCHY ENERGY BARS

12

Time: 25 minutes | Servings: 4
Serving: 1 cup
Net carbs: 11g / 0.38oz
Fiber: 8g / 0.28oz
Fat: 17g / 0.59oz
Protein: 6g / 0.21oz
Kcal: 175

INGREDIENTS:

- 5 tbsp Flaxseeds Meal
- ½ tbsp Chia Seeds
- ½ tbsp Hemp Seeds
- 5 tbsp Coconut Flakes
- ½ oz Almonds
- ½ oz Pecan Nuts
- ½ oz of Pine Nuts
- 4 tbsp Maple Syrup
- Pinch of Salt (Optional)

INSTRUCTIONS:

1. Roughly chop the nuts into small bits for an even but crunchy texture.
2. Put all the ingredients in a mixing bowl and combine them with the maple syrup. Add more syrup if necessary. Add pinch of salt to balance the sweetness.
3. Prepare a baking dish by lining some parchment paper. Spread the mixture by maintaining a half an inch thickness.
4. Bake for 20 minutes on 350°F.
5. Remove from the oven and let the mixture cool down. Chop into small pieces for munching on morning rush hours.

13

MOCHA MOUSSE

Time: 20 minutes | Servings: 4
Serving: 1
Net carbs: 6.57g / 0.23oz
Fat: 41.94g / 0.48oz
Protein: 6.03g / 0.21oz
Kcal: 421.75

INGREDIENTS:

For Cream Cheese Mixture:
- 8 oz Cream Cheese
- 3 tbsp Sour Cream
- 2 tbsp Butter
- 3 tsp Instant Coffee Powder
- 1/3 cup Stevia Erythritol blend
- 1/4 cup Cocoa Powder (Unsweetened)
- 1 ½ tsp Vanilla extract

For Whipped Cream Mixture:
- 2/3 cup Heavy Whipping Cream
- ½ tsp Vanilla extract
- 1 ½ tsp Stevia Erythritol blend

INSTRUCTIONS:

1. Put cream cheese, butter and sour cream in a mixing bowl and beat everything well with an electric mixer until a smooth consistency forms.
2. Add vanilla extract, granulated stevia erythritol blend, cocoa powder, and instant coffee powder. Mix again until everything is well incorporated.
3. Take another mixing bowl. Beat the whipping cream with a mixer until soft peaks form.
4. Add stevia erythritol and vanilla extract. Beat again.
5. Take 1/3rd of the whipped cream and slowly fold it into the cream cheese mixture. Ensure that the bubbles are not deflated. Continue the process for the remaining whipped cream.
6. 6.Transfer the mousse into small serving glasses and refrigerate for 2-3 hours before serving.

EGG BURRITO

14

Time: 7 minutes | Servings: 1
Serving: 1
Net carbs: 1g / 0.03oz
Fat: 30g / 1.06oz
Protein: 11g / 0.39oz
Kcal: 331

INGREDIENTS:

- 1 tbsp Butter
- 2 medium-sized Eggs
- 2 tbsp full-fat Cream
- Herbs & Spices (According to taste)
- Salt
- Pepper

INSTRUCTIONS:

1. In a small mixing bowl, take the eggs, cream, salt, pepper and your preferred herbs and spices. Whisk until everything is combined together.
2. Heat up the butter in a frying pan. Once the butter is melted, pour the egg mixture.
3. Spread the eggs in a circular shape by swirling the pan.
4. Cover with a lid and cook for 2 minutes.
5. Remove from the pan and put your favourite toppings.
6. Roll up the burrito. Eat right away or pack it up for lunch on the go.

15

Time: 2 minutes | Servings: 1

INGREDIENTS:

- 3/4 cup Cottage Cheese
- 3 tbsp Walnuts (Roughly Chopped)
- 1 tsp Flax Seed Oil
- 1/4 cup frozen Berries
- 1 tsp Chia Seeds

INSTRUCTIONS:

1. Place the cottage cheese in the food processor and pulse for 1-2 minutes. This will give you a lighter texture of the cheese.
2. For a thicker version, scoop up the cheese directly from the container and put it in a serving bowl.
3. Sprinkle some chia seeds and top with chopped berries. Add the walnuts and lastly, drizzle some flaxseed oil. Serve instantly.

LUNCH (15 RECIPES)

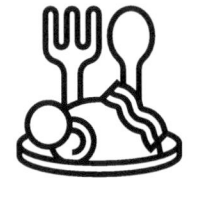

1

Time: 25 minutes | Servings: 25
Serving: 1
Net carbs: 0.9g / 0.10oz
Fat: 2.9g / 2.72oz
Protein: 2.7g / 1.59oz
kcal: 31

INGREDIENTS:

- 1 medium-sized Cauliflower (Riced)
- 3 Large Eggs
- 1 1/2 cup Cheddar Cheese (Shredded)
- 2 tsp. Paprika
- Salt and Pepper
- 1 tsp. Tumeric powder
- 3/4 tsp. dried Rosemary
- 2 tbsp. olive oil

INSTRUCTIONS:

1. Cut the cauliflower into small florets. Add them in a food processor and turn them into riced cauliflower.
2. Put it in a bowl with a little bit of water and cook in the microwave for 5 minutes. Pat dry with a kitchen towel to remove extra moisture.
3. Add one egg, shredded cheese and the spices in the cauliflower mixture. Stir a few times. Add another egg. Stir again and add the last egg. Combine everything together.
4. Scoop up some of the mixture and shape it into small patties.
5. Heat the oil in a pan over high heat. Place the patties and fry them until they are golden brown on each side.
6. Serve warm with some leafy greens.

FRIED CAULIFLOWER AND CHEESE PATTIES

CREAMED SPINACH

2

Time: 5 minutes | Servings: 1
Net carbs: 2g / 0.07oz
Fiber: 2g / 0.07oz
Fat: 26g / 0.92oz
Protein: 9g / 0.32oz
kcal: 283

INGREDIENTS:

- 3.50 oz fresh Spinach
- 2 tbsp. Cream
- 2 tbsp. Parmesan cheese (Shredded)
- 1 tbsp. Butter
- 1 tbsp. Olive Oil
- Pinch of Ground Nutmeg
- Pinch of Salt
- Pinch of Pepper

INSTRUCTIONS:

1. Heat the oil in a large pan over medium heat.
2. Once the hot is heat up, add the spinach leaves.
3. Season with some salt, pepper and the ground nutmeg.
4. Once the spinach is wilted in the pan, add the butter, cream and the cheese.
5. Cook for a minute or two while mixing everything together.
6. Turn off the stove. Serve the creamy deliciousness for a hearty vegetarian meal.

3

Time: 25 minutes | Servings: 4
Serving:1
Net carbs: 4g / 0.14oz
Fiber: 1g / 0.03oz
Fat: 11g / 0.39oz
Protein: 2g / 0.07oz
kcal: 121

INDIAN STYLE CHICKEN CURRY

INGREDIENTS:

For the Marinate
- 1 Full Chicken (Curry Cut)
- 0.35 oz Ginger Garlic Paste
- 2.12 oz Full Fat Greek Yogurt
- 1 Tsp Salt
- 1 Tsp Tumeric
- 1 Tsp Coriander Powder
- 1 Tsp Kashmiri Red Chilli Powder
- 1 Tsp Cumin Powder
- 1/2 tsp Garam Masala Powder
- 1 tsp Lime Juice

For the Curry
- 3.53 oz Onion (Finely diced)
- 4.23 oz Tomato (Finely diced)
- 1 Green Chilli
- 2 tbsp Ghee
- 1 tbsp Butter
- Chopped Coriander
- Water

INSTRUCTIONS:

1. In a mixing bowl, put all the spices and condiments for marinating and stir well to mix everything together. Place the chicken and rub each piece with the spice mixture. Once the chicken is well covered with the spices, set it aside for marinating for 2 hours.

2. Heat the ghee in a large saucepan and add in the onions. Cook the onions till they are brown. Add in 1 tbsp water and let it cook again. Repeat the process to get a dark, mushy texture.

3. Slit the green chilli in halves and add it to the onion mixture along with the diced tomatoes.

4. Add the chicken when the tomatoes melted away. Pour the water from the marinade and give everything a good stir.
5. Cook the chicken on high heat for a few minutes. Add half a cup of water and bring it to a boil. Lower the heat and cover the pan with a lid. Cook for 15-20 minutes over medium heat.
6. Add in the butter and the chopped coriander before turning off the stove. Give it another stir and serve on a bowl. Eat with keto naan or cauliflower rice to get the most of the spicy flavour.

4

Time: 20 minutes | Servings: 10
Serving: 1
Net carbs: 2.23g / 0.08oz
Fiber: 1.1g / 0.04oz
Fat: 21.8g / 0.77oz
Protein: 22.8g / 0.80oz
Kcal: 298

INGREDIENTS:

For the Salmon Patties
- 2 lb Salmon (Skinless and Cubed)
- 3/4 cup Almond Flour
- ½ cup Mayonnaise
- 2 Eggs
- 1.5 tsp Tamari Soy Sauce
- 1 tsp Lemon Zest
- ½ cup Almond Milk
- 1.5 tsp Dijon Mustard
- 1.5 tsp capers
- 1 tsp Garlic Powder
- 1 tsp Onion Powder
- 2 tsp Parsley
- Pinch of Kosher Salt
- Pinch of Pepper
- 1 tsp Avocado oil

For the Tartar Sauce
- 1/2 cup Greek Yoghurt
- ½ cup Mayonnaise
- Zest & Juice of ½ a Lemon
- 1.5 tsp Dill Relish
- 1 tsp Horseradish (Prepared)
- 1 tbsp Chives (Finely Sliced)
- Pinch of Kosher Salt
- Pinch of Pepper

INSTRUCTIONS:

1. Add all the salmon patty ingredients into a food processor and blend until all the elements are combined but remain a bit chunky. Chill the mixture in the refrigerator for 30 minutes to 3 hours.

SALMON PATTIES WITH TARTAR SAUCE

2. Heat up a large non-stick pan. Keep the heat medium-high.
3. Scoop up some of the salmon mixture and shape into small patties. Cook in the pan for 7-8 minutes until both sides turn golden brown.
4. Mix all the ingredients for the tartar sauce in a separate bowl. Serve with the warm salmon patties.

5

Time: 55 minutes | Servings: 4
Serving: 1
Net carbs: 3.4g / 0.14oz
Protein: 23.4g / 0.07oz
Fat: 48.6g / 0.25oz
Kcal: 572

INGREDIENTS:

- 5 Bacon
- 12 oz Ground Beef
- 2 tbsp Butter
- 3 cups Beef Broth
- 1/2 tsp Garlic Powder
- 1/2 tsp Onion Powder
- 2 tsp Brown Mustard
- 1 1/2 tsp Kosher Salt
- 1/2 tsp Black Pepper
- 1/2 tsp Red Pepper Flakes
- 1 tsp Cumin Powder
- 1 tsp Chili Powder
- 2 1/2 tbsp Tomato Paste
- 1 cup Shredded Cheddar Cheese
- 3 oz Cream Cheese
- 1 medium-sized Dill Pickle (Diced)
- 1/2 cup Heavy Cream

INSTRUCTIONS:

1. Cook the bacon in a frying pan until it turns crispy. Remove from the pan.
2. Add the beef to the bacon grease and cook until browned on every side.
3. Take a large pot and transfer the in it. Add butter and all the spices to cook for 30-45 seconds.
4. Add tomato paste, cheese, mustard and pickles. Pour the beef broth and cook for a few minutes.
5. Cover the pot with a lid. Cook on low heat for 20-30 minutes.
6. Remove from the pot. Serve hot with bacon and heavy cream.

BACON & CHEESEBURGER SOUP

CHEESY LETTUCE WRAPS

6

Time: 10 minutes | Servings: 1
Serving: 1
Net carbs: 3g / 0.11oz
Fiber: 8g / 0.28oz
Fat: 34g / 1.19oz
Protein: 10g / 0.35oz
kcal: 37

INGREDIENTS:

- 2 oz Lettuce Leaves
- ½ oz Butter
- ½ Avocado
- 1 medium-sized Tomato
- 1 oz shredded Mozzarella
- Salt
- Pepper

INSTRUCTIONS:

1. Chop the tomato and the avocado into cube shapes. Keep them separately.
2. Heat up a pan and melt the butter. Put the tomato cubes when the butter turns brown.
3. Put the seasoning of salt and pepper. Stir a few times.
4. Remove the tomato from the pan when they are softened up.
5. Take a lettuce leaf. Place the cooked tomato in the middle. Top with avocado and shredded mozzarella.
6. Wrap the filling with the leaf and put a toothpick to keep everything in place.
7. Serve instantly or put into your lunch box for a perfect break time snack.

7

Time: 2 minutes | Servings: 4
Serving: 1
Net carbs: 15g / 0.18oz
Fiber: 6g / 0.21oz
Fat: 3g / 0.10oz
Protein: 27g / 0.95oz
kcal: 569

INGREDIENTS:

- 12 slices of Genoa Salami
- 12 slices of Provolone
- 12 slices of Pepperoni
- 12 slices of Ham
- 6 tbsp homemade mayonnaise
- 40 black olives
- 1/2 cup Shredded Lettuce
- 2 Apples

INSTRUCTIONS:

1. Lay all the ingredients on a cutting board.
2. Slice the apples and secure them together in the shape of the apple with a rubber band.
3. Roll up the sandwich using all the ingredients except the black olives.
4. Put the sandwich, apples and the olives in a lunch box.
5. Store in the refrigerator and use within 3 days.

COBB SALAD

8

Time: 15 minutes | Servings: 1
Serving: 1
Net carbs: 2.4g / 0.08oz
Fat: 15.2g / 0.54oz
Protein: 16.7g / 0.59oz
kcal: 219

INGREDIENTS:

- ¼ cup Bacon crumbles
- 1 medium-sized Egg (Hard-boiled)
- ¼ cup Cherry Tomatoes
- 1 large Avocado
- 1 tbsp Trader Joes Organic Ranch Dressings
- 2 cups Arugula and Spinach mix

INSTRUCTIONS:

1. Prepare all the ingredients that need to be cooked or sliced up.
2. Chop the avocado into small cube shapes.
3. Place the bacon, tomatoes, arugula and spinach mix in a small container. Top with the sliced eggs, chopped avocado and finally, drizzle some salad dressing.
4. Serve instantly.

9

Time: 35 minutes | Servings: 4
Serving: 1
Net carbs: 6g / 0.21oz
Fat: 25g / 0.88oz
Protein: 66g / 2.33oz
kcal: 527

INGREDIENTS:

- 4 Chicken Breasts (Thinly Sliced)
- 2 large Eggs
- ½ cup powdered Parmesan
- 2 cups Pork Rinds (Finely Crushed)
- 1/2 cup Marinara
- 1 tsp Garlic powder
- 1/2 tsp Onion powder
- 1 cup Mozzarella Cheese (Grated)
- 1 tbsp Parsley/ Basil (Minced)

INSTRUCTIONS:

1. Preheat the oven to 350°F.
2. Take a large cookie sheet. Spray some non-stick cooking spray.
3. Beat the eggs and place the mixture on a shallow dish.
4. Mix the powdered parmesan, pork rinds, onion powder and garlic powder. Put the mixture in another shallow dish.
5. Dip the chicken breast slices into the egg mixture. Cover them with the pork rind mixture. Repeat the process again so that the chicken is well-covered in every side.
6. Bake the chicken breast slices for 15-20 minutes until the temperature of the chicken reaches 160°F.

7. Remove from the oven and spread the marinara over the chicken slices.
8. Sprinkle with mozzarella and bake for another 5 minutes. The temperature needs to be 165°F.
9. Serve hot with sprinkles of minced herbs on top.

10

Time: 30 minutes | Servings: 2
Serving: 1
Net carbs: 4.7g / 1.66oz
Fat: 16.8g / 0.59oz
Protein: 2.3g / 0.08oz
Fiber: 1.1g / 0.04oz
kcal: 180

INGREDIENTS:

- 2 large Tomatoes
- 2 tbsp Olive Oil
- 1 tbsp Shallot (Chopped)
- 1 clove of Garlic
- 1 tsp Dried Oregano
- 1 tsp Dried Mint
- 1 tbsp Fresh Peppermint
- 1 tbsp Feta Cheese
- ½ cup Zucchini
- ½ tbsp Pine Nuts
- ¼ tsp Salt
- 1/8 tsp Black Pepper Powder

INSTRUCTIONS:

1. Slice the tops of the tomatoes and carefully remove the center.
2. Preheat the oven to 360°F.
3. Chop the zucchini into small cubes
4. Heat olive oil in a large pan over medium heat. Add onion and garlic and cook until tender.
5. Add the zucchini, chopped tomato pulp, oregano and mint. Season with salt and pepper.
6. Add the crumbled feta cheese when the zucchini becomes tender. Stir well and remove from the pan.
7. Put the mixture in two tomatoes and cover with the tomato tops.
8. Bake for 20-25 minutes.
9. Remove the tops and sprinkle the pine nuts. Serve hot.

STUFFED TOMATOES

ZUCCHINI BOLOGNESE

11

Time: 9 hours | Servings: 6
Serving: 1
Net carbs: 6g / 0.21oz
Fat: 28.7g / 1.01oz
Protein: 29g / 1.02oz
kcal: 402

INGREDIENTS:

For the Zucchini Noodles
- 20 oz Zucchini
- 2 tbsp Olive Oil
- 1 cup shredded Mozzarella Cheese
- Pinch of Salt
- Pinch of Pepper

For the Bolognese Sauce
- 1.5 oz Ground Beef
- ¼ cup Chicken Bouillon (Prepared)
- 3.5oz Onion (Diced)
- 1 tbsp Olive Oil
- 3 cloves of Garlic (Minced)
- ½ tsp ground Nutmeg
- ½ tsp Thyme
- ½ tsp ground Marjoram
- 2 tbsp Heavy Whipping Cream
- 2 cups Marinara Sauce
- Salt and Pepper (To taste)

INSTRUCTIONS:

1. Heat up the olive oil in a frying pan. Add the onion and cook until they turn translucent.
2. Add the minced garlic. Put the ground beef when the garlic turns brownish.
3. Add the thyme, nutmeg, marjoram, salt and pepper. Mix everything together and cook until the beef turns brown.

4. Add the marinara sauce, heavy whipping cream and chicken bouillon.
5. Turn off the heat off and allow it to rest for 10 minutes.
6. Put the mixture in a slow cooker and cover with a lid. Cook for about 8 hours.
7. Make some zucchini noodles using a vegetable spiralizer. Season with olive oil, salt and pepper. Put it in a casserole dish.
8. Top first with the bolognese sauce, then with the mozzarella cheese.
9. Bake for 15-20 minutes at 350°F and serve hot.

STEAMED PORK CABBAGE ROLLS

12

Time: 30 minutes | Servings: 8
Serving: 1
Net carbs: 1.86g / 0.06oz
Fat: 12.67g / 0.45oz
Protein: 17.05g / 0.60oz
Kcal: 191.6

INGREDIENTS:

For the Rolls
- 8 medium-sized cabbage leaves
- 2 stalks Green Onion (Thinly Sliced)
- 1 oz ground Pork
- 1 medium-sized Egg
- 1 tsp Ginger (Grated)
- 2 tbsp Soy Sauce

For the Dipping Sauce
- 1/4 cup Soy Sauce
- 1/4 tsp Salt
- 2 tsp Sriracha Sauce
- 1/2 tsp Erythritol

INSTRUCTIONS:

1. Boil water in a large pot. Add the cabbage leaves when the water is boiling.
2. Carefully remove the cabbage leaves when they soften up.
3. Take a large mixing bowl. Add ground pork, egg, green onion, ginger and soy sauce. Combine everything together.
4. Place about 2 tbsp of the pork mixture into a cabbage leaf. Roll

the leaf like a burrito.
5. Repeat the process for the remaining cabbage leaves.
6. Place the rolls in a steamer and cook for 20-25 minutes until the pork is cooked.
7. Mix the soy sauce, sriracha sauce, salt and erythritol. Put the dipping sauce in a small dish.
8. Serve the hot rolls with the mouth-smacking dipping sauce.

AVOCADO & EGG SALAD BOWL

13

Time: 10 minutes | Servings: 2
Serving: 1
Net carbs: 2g / 0.07oz
Fat: 51g / 1.79oz
Protein: 20g / 0.70oz
Fiber: 5g / 0.18oz
kcal: 575

INGREDIENTS:

For the Rolls
- 6 medium-sized Eggs
- 1 medium-sized Avocado
- 1/3 cup homemade Mayonnaise
- 1 tsp Dijon Mustard
- ½ tsp Lemon Juice
- Pinch of Salt
- Pinch of Pepper
- 1/8 tsp dill
- ½ tbsp Chopped Parsley

INSTRUCTIONS:

1. Prepare 6 hard-boiled eggs using your favourite method.
2. Place the eggs in an ice bath right away in order to prevent further cooking.
3. Smash the eggs, season with salt and pepper and place them in a serving bowl.
4. Mash the avocado in a separate bowl and season with salt and pepper.
5. Combine all the ingredients together. Chill in the refrigerator for 30 minutes for a refreshing salad bowl.
6. Serve with chopped parsley on top.

14

Time: 60 minutes | Servings: 6
Serving: 1
Net carbs: 2g / 0.07oz
Fat: 47g / 1.66oz
Protein: 20g / 0.70oz
Kcal: 517

INGREDIENTS:

- 8 large Eggs
- 10 oz Bacon
- 1 cup Cream
- 1 cup Mozzarella Cheese (Grated)
- 1 tsp Salt
- 1 tsp Pepper

INSTRUCTIONS:

1. Preheat the oven to 356°F. Grease a baking pan with non-stick cooking spray.
2. Fry the bacon until they are cooked halfway through.
3. Whisk the eggs and cream with salt and pepper. Mix other herbs of your choice if you feel like altering the taste.
4. Place the bacon and half of the grated cheese into the mixture.
5. Pour the mixture in the baking dish.
6. Sprinkle the remaining cheese on top.
7. Bake for 40 - 45 minutes until the top turns golden brown.
8. Remove from oven and cut into 6 slices.
9. Serve when it cools down.

LUNCHBOX OMELETTE

LUNCHBOX OMELETTE

15

Time: 10 minutes | Servings: 1
Serving: 1 bowl
Net carbs: 4g / 0.14oz
Fiber: 1g / 0.03oz
Fat: 38g / 1.34oz
Protein: 22g / 0.78oz
Kcal: 444

INGREDIENTS:

- 1 large Tomato
- 3.20 oz Buffalo Mozzarella Cheese
- 2 tbsp. Pine Nuts

Pesto

- 1 oz Parmesan cheese
- 1 1/2 tbsp. Pine Nuts
- 1 tsp. Fresh Garlic
- 2 tbsp. Parsley
- 3 1/5 tbsp. Basil
- 3/4 cup Extra Virgin Olive Oil
- ½ tsp. Lemon/Lime Juice
- Pinch of Salt

INSTRUCTIONS:

1. To prepare the pesto, grate the cheese and put it in the blender along with the garlic and the pine nuts. Blend until a semi-smooth texture forms.
2. Add in the rest of the ingredients required for the pesto and blend for a smooth consistency.
3. Once the pesto is done, you can store in the fridge for using in other Italian recipes including pasta and pizza.
4. For the salad, chop the tomato and the cheese into small cube shapes and place them in a mixing bowl.
5. Add the pine nuts and 1 tbsp. pesto in the mixture.
6. Give it a good stir and serve as a healthy salad dish.

DINNER (15 RECIPES)

MASHED CAULIFLOWER

1

Time: 15 minutes | Servings: 4
Serving: 1
Net carb: 5.64g / 0.19oz
Fiber: 5.25g / 0.19oz
Fat: 5.5g / 0.19oz
Protein: 6.5g / 0.23g
Kcal: 113.5

INGREDIENTS:

- 1 large Cauliflower
- 4 Garlic cloves
- 1 tbsp unsalted butter
- ¼ cup grated Parmesan
- Kosher Salt
- Ground Pepper

INSTRUCTIONS:

1. Chop the cauliflower head into small florets.
2. Boil water in a large pot. Season the water with 1 tbsp of salt. Add the cauliflower florets and the garlic cloves. Boil until the cauliflower softens up for mashing with ease.
3. Strain the garlic and the cauliflower while keeping 1 cup of the boiling water for later use.
4. Put all the ingredients required for the recipe into a blender. Add a bit of the reserved water if necessary. Blend until you get a thick, smooth and creamy texture.
5. Add salt, pepper or other spices or herbs according to your preference.
6. Serve right away or store in the refrigerator up to 5 days.

2

Time: 4 hours | Servings: 5
Serving: 1
Net carb: 4.42g / 1.16oz
Fat: 17.5g / 0.62oz
Protein: 29.99g / 1.06oz
Kcal: 297.2

INGREDIENTS:

- 1 lb Chicken Tenders
- 24 oz Button Mushrooms
- 8 slices Bacon (Chopped and Cooked)
- 3 Garlic cloves
- ½ tsp dried Basil
- ¼ tsp dried Thyme
- ½ tsp dried Oregano
- 1 cup Chicken Broth
- 2 Bay leaves
- 2 tbsp Butter
- ¼ cup Heavy Whipping Cream
- ¼ cup Parsley (Chopped)
- Salt
- Pepper

INSTRUCTIONS:

1. Wash the mushrooms and remove the stems.
2. Cut the chicken tenders into small bite-size pieces.
3. Turn on the stove and set a slow cooker. Place the mushrooms first and let it soften up a bit.
4. Add all the ingredients except the butter and heavy whipping cream. Cover with a lid and cook for 3-4 hours on low heat.
5. Before you turn off the stove, add the butter and the cream. Stir a few times to mix everything together.
6. Serve hot with bacon and chopped parsley on top.

CHICKEN & MUSHROOM STEW

BUFFALO CHICKEN SOUP

3

Time: 35 minutes | Servings: 8
Serving: 1 ½ Cups
Net carbs: 5g / 0.18oz
Fat: 53g / 1.87oz
Protein: 32g / 1.13oz
Fiber: 1g / 0.03oz
kcal: 630

INGREDIENTS:

- 1 Rotisserie Chicken (Cooked and Shredded)
- 3 cups Cheddar Cheese
- 2 tbsp Butter
- 4 ribs Celery (Chopped)
- 6 cups Chicken Broth
- 1 tbsp Chopped Onion
- 3 cloves of Garlic (Chopped)
- 2 tbsp Ranch Dressing Mix
- 2 cups Heavy Cream
- 2/3 cup Hot Sauce
- Blue Cheese (Optional)

INSTRUCTIONS:

1. Heat up the butter in a skillet.
2. Add the celery, onion and garlic and saute until they turn tender and translucent.
3. Take a stockpot. Add the chicken broth and cook over medium heat for 2 minutes.
4. Add the sauteed veggies, shredded chicken, hot sauce and ranch dressing mix. Let it simmer for 15 minutes.
5. Reduce the heat. Add cream and cheese right before serving.
6. Stir everything together.
7. Serve hot with crumbled blue cheese on top.

4

Time: 25 minutes | Servings: 8
Serving: 1
Net carbs: 6.5g / 0.23oz
Fiber: 4.5g / 0.14oz
Fat: 14.5g / 0.51oz
Protein: 9g / 0.32oz
Kcal: 190

INGREDIENTS:

- 2 cup Almond Flour
- 4 Egg Whites
- 2 Egg Yolks
- 2 tsp Baking Powder
- 3 tbsp Psyllium husk powder
- 1/2 tsp Xanthan Gum
- 1/2 cup Hot Water
- 1 tsp Sesame Seeds
- Pinch of Salt

INSTRUCTIONS:

1. Preheat the oven to 356°F.
2. Beat the egg whites to form stiff peaks.
3. Whisk the egg yolks in a separate bowl until they turn pale and almost double in size.
4. In a medium-sized mixing bowl, add the almond flour, baking powder, psyllium husk powder and xanthan gum.
5. Add the dry mixture into the egg mixtures. Add hot water and blend everything together.
6. Take some olive oil in your hands. Knead the dough and separate 8 portions. Roll the dough into 8 ball-size pieces. Press lightly on the balls so that they form an oval shape. Cut a cross on the bread and sprinkle sesame seeds.
7. Place them on a prepared baking dish and bake for 25-30 miutes.
8. Remove from the oven when the bread turns brown in the middle.

CRUNCHY BREAD ROLLS

EGGPLANT PARMESAN

5

Time: 20 minutes | Servings: 4
Serving: 1
Net carbs: 5g / 0.18oz
Fiber: 4g / 0.14oz
Fat: 18g / 0.63oz
Protein: 14g / 0.67oz
Kcal: 241

INGREDIENTS:

- 10.5 oz Eggplant
- 5 oz Fresh Buffalo Mozzarella
- 7 oz Marinara Sauce
- 1.5 oz Parmesan Cheese
- Pinch of Salt

INSTRUCTIONS:

1. Slice the eggplant into half-inch thickness. Sprinkle salt and leave for 30 minutes.
2. Pat the eggplant slices with a paper towel to reduce the extra moisture. Fry the eggplant in a pan or grill them in the oven.
3. Take an ovenproof dish. Layer with the marinara sauce and parmesan cheese. Add a layer of eggplant and top with half of the mozzarella cheese. Add another layer of eggplant, marinara sauce and sprinkle the remaining mozzarella cheese.
4. Bake for 15-20 minutes at 350°F until the top turns golden brown.
5. Serve hot.

6

TUNA SALAD

Time: 20 minutes | Servings: 1
Serving: 1
Net carbs: 1g / 0.03oz
Fiber: 2g / 0.07oz
Fat: 23g / 0.81oz
Protein: 21g / 0.74oz
kcal: 298

INGREDIENTS:

- 1 canned tuna
- 2 slices of Bacon
- 1 large Egg
- 1 tbsp homemade Mayonnaise
- 1 tbsp chopped Onion
- 2 tsp Dijon Mustard
- Pinch of Pepper
- 1 tbsp Sour cream
- 1/4 tsp dill

INSTRUCTIONS:

1. Boil the egg and chop it into small pieces.
2. Cook the bacon until it is crisp.
3. Drain the tuna and put it in a bowl.
4. Add the chopped onion and the chopped egg.
5. Mix with the ground pepper, mayonnaise, mustard and sour cream.
6. Top with the crumbled bacon.
7. Sprinkle some dill and serve.

PORK CHOPS WITH CARAMELIZED ONION

7

Time: 60 minutes | Servings: 4
Serving: 1
Net carbs: 6.3g / 0.22oz
Fiber: 1.02g / 0.03oz
Fat: 18.23g / 0.64oz
Protein: 36.98g / 1.30oz
kcal: 352

INGREDIENTS:

- 6 slices of Bacon
- 1 large Onion (Thinly Sliced)
- 4 Pork Chops (1-inch thick, Bone-in)
- 1/2 cup Chicken Broth
- 1/4 cup Heavy Cream
- Salt and Pepper (To taste)

INSTRUCTIONS:

1. Cook the bacon in a large skillet over medium heat. Remove from the pan when they turn crisp.
2. Add sliced onions to the bacon grease. Season with salt and pepper. Cook for 15-20 minutes until the onions become golden brown.
3. Remove the onions from the skillet and add to the bacon in a bowl.
4. Increase the heat to medium-high. Add the pork chops in the pan.
5. Sprinkle salt and pepper and cook for 10-15 minutes on both sides. Remove from the pan when the internal temperature of the pork chops reaches 135°F.
6. Add the chicken broth and cream to the pan and let it simmer for 2-3 minutes.
7. Add the onion and bacon mixture to the pan and stir everything to combine well.
8. Serve the pork chops in a plate and top with the caramelized onions and bacon bits.

8

Time: 60 minutes | Servings: 6
Serving: 1
Net carbs: 4g / 0.14oz
Fiber: 2g / 0.07oz
Fat: 29g / 1.02oz
Protein: 33g / 1.16oz
kcal: 344

INGREDIENTS:

- 2 lb Ground Beef
- 2 Large Eggs
- 1/4 cup Yeast
- 1/2 tbsp Kosher Salt
- 1 tsp Ground Pepper
- 2 tbsp Olive Oil
- 1/4 cup Parsley (Minced)
- 4 cloves Garlic (Minced)
- 1 tbsp Lemon Zest
- 1/4 cup Dried Oregano

INSTRUCTIONS:

1. Preheat the oven to 400°F.
2. Take a large mixing bowl. Break the ground beef and add the yeast, salt and pepper. Stir until they are combined well.
3. Add the eggs, avocado oil, parsley, oregano and garlic in a food processor. Pulse a few times until the eggs turn frothy.
4. Mix the eggs and the beef together.
5. Grease an 8×4 loaf pan and put the beef mixture.
6. Bake for about an hour or so until the top becomes golden brown.
7. Remove from the oven and drain all the excess fluid.
8. Let the meatloaf rest for about 10 minutes.
9. Slice into 6 pieces. Serve with lemon zest sprinkled on top.

OVEN-BAKED MEATLOAF

CHICKEN & GREEN BEANS ALMONDINE

9

Time: 25 minutes | Servings: 4
Serving: 1
Net carbs: 11g / 0.39oz
Fat: 18g / 0.56oz
Protein: 31g / 1.09oz
Fiber: 3g / 0.10oz
kcal: 321

INGREDIENTS:

- 1 lb Chicken Breast/ Chicken Thighs
- 1 lb Green Beans
- 2 tbsp Olive Oil
- 1/3 cup Almonds (Thinly Sliced)
- 1 tbsp Garlic (Minced)

For the Seasoning

- 1 tbsp Olive Oil
- 1 1/2 tsp Cumin Powder
- 1 1/2 tsp Onion Powder
- 1 1/2 tsp Garlic Powder
- 1 tbsp Dried Rosemary
- Pinch of Sea Salt
- Pinch of Pepper

INSTRUCTIONS:

1. Steam the green beans in a steamer basket. Remove after 5 minutes or so when the beans turn soft and tender.
2. Put them in an ice bath to prevent cooking further.
3. Mix all the seasoning in a mixing bowl. Rub each chicken piece with the seasoning.
4. Heat up some olive oil in a non-stick skillet. then toss add the chicken. Add the chicken and cook for 6-8 minutes over medium heat. Remove from the pan when the chicken turns golden brown.

5. Reduce the heat and add the minced garlic and sliced almonds. Add the green beans when the almonds become brownish. Cook for a minute or two over medium heat.
6. Remove from the pan and serve with the cooked chicken.

SALISBURY STEAK IN SLOW COOKER

10

Time: 25 minutes | Servings: 4
Serving: 1
Net carbs: 6g / 0.28oz
Fat: 18g / 0.63oz
Protein: 32g / 1.13oz
kcal: 332

INGREDIENTS:

- 2 lbs Ground Beef
- 1/2 cup Beef Broth/ Plain Water
- 1 large Egg
- 1 12 oz Beef Gravy
- 1/2 cup Breadcrumbs
- 1/4 cup Milk
- 8 oz Mushrooms (Sliced)
- 1 small Onion(Sliced)
- 1 tsp Onion Powder
- 1 tsp Garlic Powder
- 1 tbsp Olive Oil
- 1 tsp Salt
- 1/2 tsp Black Pepper
- 1 tbsp Cornstarch
- 2 tbsp Parsley (Chopped)
- 2 tbsp Water

INSTRUCTIONS:

1. Take the ground beef, beaten egg, milk, breadcrumbs, onion powder, garlic powder, salt and black pepper in a large mixing bowl. Shape the mixture into 6 patties.
2. Heat the olive oil. Add the patties when the oil is hot and cook for 10-12 minutes until both sides turn golden brown. Keep the heat over medium-high during the process.
3. Take a slow cooker and add the mushrooms and onion. Place the beef patties on top.
4. Pour the beef gravy and beef broth/ plain water into the cooker. Cover with a lid. Decrease the heat to low and cook for 4-6 hours.

5. Take out the patties and cover them with a foil paper to maintain the temperature.
6. Mix the cornstarch with 2 tbsp of water and pour the mixture into the slow cooker.
7. Cook for 3-5 minutes on high heat until the sauce thickens up.
8. Serve the patties on a dish and spoon the sauce on top. Garnish with some chopped parsley.

MEXICAN STYLE CAULIFLOWER RICE

11

Time: 25 minutes | Servings: 4
Serving: 1
Net carbs: 7g / 0.25oz
Fiber: 4g / 0.14oz
Fat: 7g / 0.25oz
Protein: 4g / 0.14oz
kcal: 117

INGREDIENTS:

- 1 large Cauliflower
- 2 tbsp. Olive Oil
- ¼ cup Onion (Chopped)
- 2 tbsp Tomato Puree
- 1 Jalapeno (Minced)
- ½ cup Chicken/Beef broth
- 1 Garlic clove (Minced)
- Pinch of Turmeric Powder
- 1 tsp Chili Powder
- Pinch of Salt
- Pinch of Pepper
- 1 tbsp Sour cream
- Chopped Cilantro
- 1 tbsp cubed Tomatoes

INSTRUCTIONS:

1. Chop the cauliflower head into small florets and grate them into tiny bits in a food processor.
2. Heat up the olive oil in a large skillet. Add the tomato puree and stir everything together.
3. Add the chopped onion and minced jalapeno. Cook for 3-5 minutes.
4. Pour the broth when the ingredients softens up a bit. Stir for 2 minutes.
5. Add the riced cauliflower and season with salt, pepper, turmeric powder and chili powder. Ensure that everything is evenly coated with the spices.

6. Check for the kick of the spices. Add more jalapeno if necessary.
7. Cook for 15 minutes and remove from the skillet when the cauliflower softens.
8. Serve hot with the sour cream, cubed tomatoes and chopped cilantro on top.

SHRIMP ALFREDO

12

Time: 15 minutes | Servings: 4
Serving: 1
Net carbs: 6.51g / 0.23oz
Fat: 17.55g / 0.62oz
Protein: 22.93g / 0.81oz
kcal: 297.83

INGREDIENTS:

- 1 lb raw Shrimp
- 1 tbsp Butter
- 4 oz Cream Cheese (Cubed)
- ½ cup Parmesan Cheese (Shredded)
- ½ cup Whole Milk
- 1 tbsp Garlic Powder
- 5 small-sized Tomatoes (Thinly Sliced)
- 1 tsp Dried Basil
- 1 tsp Salt
- ¼ cup Kale

INSTRUCTIONS:

1. Heat up the butter in a large skillet.
2. Add the shrimp and cook over low heat.
3. Add the tomatoes and the cream cheese cubes when the shrimp turns slightly pink.
4. Pour milk after a minute or two. Turn the heat to medium. Stir continuously so that the cream cheese completely melts into the milk.

5. Sprinkle the seasoning of salt, garlic amd basil. Stir again.
6. Put the parmesan cheese and let everything simmer for a while.
7. Add kale when the sauce thickens up.
8. Give everything a good stir and remove from the pan. Serve hot with a keto bread on the side.

SHRIMP ALFREDO

13

Time: 20 minutes | Servings: 4
Serving: 1
Net carbs: 7g / 0.25oz
Fat: 27g / 0.95oz
Protein: 12g / 0.43oz
kcal: 318

INGREDIENTS:

- 16 oz Tofu
- 2 medium-sized Bell Peppers
- 1 tbsp Tomato Puree
- 2 tbsp Coconut Oil
- 1 15 oz Coconut Milk
- 1 tsp Thai Curry Paste
- 2 tsp Chili Flakes
- 1 Garlic clove (Minced)
- ½ tsp Ginger (Minced)
- 1 tbsp Almond Butter
- 1 stalk Lemongrass
- 1/4 cup Soy Sauce

INSTRUCTIONS:

1. Chop the tofu into small cubes.
2. Slice the bell peppers into thin strips.
3. Heat up the coconut oil over medium heat.
4. Add bell pepper, garlic, ginger and lemongrass (cut into 3 pieces).
5. Pour in the coconut milk after a minute. Sprinkle the chili flakes. Stir everything together.
6. Add the soy sauce, curry paste, tomato paste and almond butter when the coconut milk thickens up a bit.
7. Put in the tofu cubes after a minute. Cook over medium heat for 15 minutes until the sauce turns thick.
8. Serve hot with cauliflower rice.

14

Time: 20 minutes | Servings: 4
Serving: 1
Net carbs: 12g / 0.42oz
Fat: 8g / 0.28oz
Protein: 2g / 0.07oz
kcal: 226

INGREDIENTS:

- 1 cup Broccoli Florets
- 1 tbsp Sesame Oil
- 1/8 cup Soy Sauce
- 1/2 Green Pepper (Chopped)
- 1 bunch Asparagus
- 1/2 Red Pepper (Chopped)
- 1/2 cup Onion (Chopped)
- 2 cloves of Garlic (Minced)
- 1 tbsp Ginger (Grated)

INSTRUCTIONS:

1. Heat up the sesame oil in a large skillet. Keep the heat over medium-high.
2. Add the veggies, minced garlic and grated ginger when the oil is hot enough. Stir everything and cook for 4 to 5 minutes.
3. Pour the soy sauce when the vegetables soften up.
4. Cook for a minute or two.
5. Serve with keto cauliflower rice.

CREAMY GARLIC MUSHROOMS

15

Time: 40 minutes | Servings: 8
Serving: 1
Net carbs: 7g / 0.25oz
Fat: 35g / 1.23oz
Protein: 11g / 0.39oz
kcal: 387

INGREDIENTS:

- 8 oz Bacon
- 26 oz Button Mushrooms
- 2 tbsp Butter
- 1/4 cup White Wine/ Chicken Stock
- 1 1/2 cups Heavy Cream
- 1 tbsp Olive Oil
- 6 cloves of Garlic (Chopped)
- 1/2 cup shredded Mozzarella
- 1 tbsp Parsley (Chopped)
- 1 tsp Thyme (Chopped)
- 1/4 cup shredded Parmesan Cheese
- Salt and Pepper (To Taste)

INSTRUCTIONS:

1. Cut the bacon into thin strips.
2. Fry the bacon over medium heat until they turn crispy. Set aside.
3. Melt the butter in the bacon grease. When the butter melts down completely, add the mushrooms and olive oil. Cook for 2-3 minutes until the mushrooms appear brownish.
4. Pour in the white wine or the chicken stock. Keep stirring. Let it simmer for 2-3 minutes.

5. Preheat your oven to 350°F at this point.
6. Add the garlic in the mushroom mixture. Stir in the cream, parsley, thyme, salt and pepper after a minute.
7. Reduce the heat to low. Let it simmer for 4-5 minutes until the sauce thickens up.
8. Add the cooked bacon in the mixture. Stir everything and remove from the pan.
9. Place the mixture in an oven-proof dish. Top with mozzarella and shredded parmesan.
10. Bake for 3-5 minutes until the cheese has melted.
11. Serve hot with a keto bread on the side.

SNACKS & DESSERTS (8 RECIPES)

1

Time: 25 minutes | Servings: 6
Serving: 1
Net Carb: 3.2g / 0.11oz
Fat: 27g / 0.95oz
Protein: 18.2g / 0.64oz
Kcal: 335

INGREDIENTS:

Crust
- 8 oz. Mozzarella Cheese (2 cups)
- 3/4 cup Almond Flour
- 3 tbsp. Cream Cheese
- 1 tbsp. Psyllium Husk Powder
- 1 large Egg
- 1/2 tsp. Salt
- 1/2 tsp. Pepper
- 1 tbsp. Italian Seasoning

Toppings
- 4 oz. Mozzarella Cheese (1 cup)
- 1/2 cup Tomato Sauce (unsweetened)
- Sliced Pepperoni (12-16 pieces)
- Dried Oregano (optional)

INSTRUCTIONS:

1. Prepare the mozzarella for the base by melting it in the microwave. Once it's melted and have cooled down to the room temperature, add all the other ingredients (except olive oil) to form a dough.

PEPPERONI PIZZA

2. Knead the pizza dough into a ball shape. Spread olive oil all over the ball and gently press on it to form a circular shape. The thickness should be half an inch or less according to your preference.

3. Bake the crust in 400°F for about 10 minutes. Flip the crust and bake for 3 or 4 minutes.

4. Remove from the oven and spread all your favourite toppings. Just to blend everything together, bake for another 5 minutes.

5. Serve warm.

2

Time: 20 minutes | Servings: 4
Serving: 1
Net carbs: 2.9g / 0.10oz
Fat: 8.05g / 0.28oz
Protein: 2.18g / 0.08
kcal: 86.94

INGREDIENTS:

- 5 oz. low-carb Milk Chocolate
- 3 large Eggs
- 4 tbsp. unsweetened Cocoa Powder
- ½ cup Swerve Confectioner's Sweetener
- 4 tbsp. melted butter
- ¼ cup Mascarpone Cheese
- ½ tsp. Salt

INSTRUCTIONS:

1. Take a large mixing bowl. Beat the eggs and the sweetener for 3-5 minutes until a pale, frothy mixture forms.
2. Add the cheese and beat again till you get a smooth texture.
3. Sift in the salt and half of the cocoa powder and mix slowly. Add the remaining cocoa powder and mix again. Once everything is dissolved, your batter is ready and you can start on the chocolate.
4. Break the chocolate into small pieces and put them in a glass bowl. Microwave the chocolate until it is completely melted. In order to ensure a fast and effective outcome, stir the mixture every once in a while during the melting process.
5. Add the butter and stir for an even mixture. When it's cooled a bit, fold the chocolate into the prepared batter. Stir till a smooth texture forms.

FLOURLESS BROWNIES

FLOURLESS BROWNIES

6. Heat the oven to 375°F and line a 8x8 baking pan with parchment paper.
7. Pour the batter in the pan and bake for 25 minutes.
8. Remove from the oven and cut into small pieces after it cools down.

3

Time: 5 minutes | Servings: 1
Serving: 1
Net carbs: 4g / 0.14oz
Fat: 11g / 0.39oz
Fiber: 7gm / 0.25oz
Protein: 15g / 0.53oz
Kcal: 215

INGREDIENTS:

- 2 large Eggs
- 2 tbsp. Coconut flour
- 1/2 tsp. Baking powder
- 1 tsp. unsweetened Cocoa powder
- 1/2 tbsp. Instant Espresso
- 1 tsp Vanilla Extract
- 2 1/2 tbsp. Granulated Erythritol

Cake Topping:
- 1 tsp. melted Coconut oil
- 2 tbsp. unsweetened Chocolate Chips

INSTRUCTIONS:

1. In a small mixing bowl, add all the dry ingredients. Stir the ingredients together.
2. Add in the eggs and the other wet ingredients in a separate bowl and mix them well.
3. Combine all the ingredients together and stir a few times until a smooth texture forms.
4. Pour the batter in a large mug and microwave for 1-2 minutes.
5. Add the topping in a small bowl and microwave them until they melt.
6. Pour the chocolate glaze on top the mug cake and enjoy while it's warm and soft.

KETO MICROWAVE MUG CAKE

PIZZA CHIPS

4

Time: 5 minutes | Servings: 21
Serving: 1
Net carbs: 0.16g / 0.005oz
Fat: 5.3g / 0.19oz
Protein: 3g / 0.11oz
Kcal: 61.29

INGREDIENTS:

- 6 oz sliced pepperoni
- 5.25 oz mozzarella cheese (shredded)

INSTRUCTIONS:

1. Preheat the oven to 400°F.
2. Spread the pepperonis in small diamond shapes (in batches of 4) on 2/3 cookie sheets.
3. Bake them for 5 minutes so that they are greasy and semi crispy.
4. Sprinkle the shredded cheese on top and bake for another 2-3 minutes until the cheese is crisp and melted.
5. Put them on a paper towel to soak up extra grease. Serve hot with marinara sauce.

5

Time: 5 minutes | Servings: 6
Serving: 4 Breadsticks
Net carbs: 3.6g / 0.13oz
Fat: 24.7g / 0.87oz
Protein: 12.8g / 0.45oz
kcal: 314

INGREDIENTS:

- 8 oz Mozzarella Cheese
- 3/4 cup Almond Flour
- 3 tbsp. Cream Cheese
- 1 tbsp. Psyllium Husk Powder
- 1 tsp. Baking Powder
- 1 large Egg
- 1 tsp. Garlic Powder
- 1 Tsp. onion powder
- ¼ cup Parmesan cheese
- 3 oz Cheddar Cheese

INSTRUCTIONS:

1. Preheat the oven to 400°F.
2. Mix the egg and the cream cheese and set aside.
3. In a separate bowl, mix almond flour, psyllium husk powder and baking powder.
4. Melt the mozzarella cheese in the microwave. Put the dry and the wet ingredients into the melted cheese.
5. Knead the dough and flatten it into a half an inch thick crust.
6. Spread a mixture of parmesan cheese, cheddar cheese, garlic powder and onion powder on top.
7. Cut into breadstick sizes and put them in the oven.
8. Bake for 13-15 minutes and serve hot.

COCONUT CASHEW BARS

6

Time: 8 minutes | Servings: 8
Serving: 1
Net carbs: 4.45g / 0.16oz
Fat: 18.39g / 0.65oz
Protein: 4.55g / 0.16oz
kcal: 197.36

INGREDIENTS:

- 1 cup Almond Flour
- ¼ cup Shredded Coconut (Unsweetened)
- ¼ cup Butter (Melted)
- ¼ cup sugar-free Maple Syrup
- ½ cup Cashews (Raw or Roasted)
- 1 tsp. Cinnamon Powder
- Pinch of salt

INSTRUCTIONS:

1. Put the melted butter and the almond flour in a mixing bowl and mix them well.
2. Add cinnamon powder, salt, maple syrup and coconut in the mixture. Whisk a few times.
3. Roughly chop up the cashew nuts and add them into the dough. Mix well.
4. Prepare a baking dish by lining with parchment paper.
5. Spread the dough in the dish in an even layer and put them in the refrigerator.
6. Remove the coconut cashew mixture after 2 hours or more. Slice it into 8 bars and enjoy with a cup of hot tea!

7

Time: 10 minutes | Servings: 1
Serving: 1
Net carbs: 5g / 0.18oz
Fat: 22g / 0.77oz
Protein: 10g / 0.35oz
kcal: 250

INGREDIENTS:

- 3.50 oz White Mushrooms
- 1.75 oz Oyster Mushrooms
- 1 tbsp. Butter
- 1 sprig of Rosemary
- 1 clove of Garlic (Minced)
- 1 tsp. Olive Oil
- Pinch of Salt
- Pinch of Pepper

INSTRUCTIONS:

1. Heat the olive oil in a pan over medium heat.
2. Add in both the mushrooms. Stir a few times and season with salt and pepper.
3. Add half of the butter and the rosemary sprig. After a minute, put all the minced garlic.
4. Turn off the stove when the garlic turns brown. Pour the remaining butter and give everything a good stir.
5. Serve hot with a piece of keto bread.

SAUTEED MUSHROOMS

TORTILLA CHIPS

8

Time: 45 minutes | Servings: 6
Serving: 1
Net carbs: 7.3g / 0.26oz
Fiber: 6.7g / 0.24oz
Fat: 4g / 0.14oz
Protein: 11.3g / 0.40oz
kcal: 112

INGREDIENTS:

- 1/2 cup Chia Seeds
- 4 Egg whites
- Pinch of Salt
- 1 cup Water

INSTRUCTIONS:

1. Preheat the oven to 350°F.
2. Line a baking pan with silicone baking mat.
3. Put all the ingredients in a food processor and blend until a smooth mixture forms.
4. Spread the blended mixture in the pan. Try to ensure that the layer is as even as possible.
5. Bake for 35-40 minutes.
6. Remove from the oven when the center is hard and crispy.
7. Break into small pieces for bite-size tortilla chips.
8. Store in a plastic zip-top bag or an air-tight container. Grab a handful whenever you feel like snacking.

By maintaining a balanced keto meal plan, it is very easy to lose weight within a short time. If you are interested to know how, check out our expertly curated daily meal plan in the next section.

DAY 1

BREAKFAST

Sausage & Egg Breakfast Bowl (Serves 1/7 min)

Serving: 1
Net carbs: 2g / 0.07oz
Fat: 59g / 2.08oz
Protein: 25g / 0.88oz
kcal: 649

INGREDIENTS:

- 1/4 cup Sausage
- 2 whole Eggs
- 2 tbs Butter
- 1 tbsp Cheddar Cheese
- Salt & Pepper (To Taste)

INSTRUCTIONS:

1. Cook the sausages until they are crisp and crumbled.
2. Crack the eggs in a bowl. Scramble with a fork. Season with salt and pepper.
3. Add 1 tbsp of butter on a non-stick pan over medium-high heat.
4. Add the eggs in the pan when the butter has melted. Stir inwards so that the egg is nicely scrambled.
5. Place the remaining butter in the middle and melt it with the cooking eggs.
6. Add the cheese and the sausages when the eggs turn glossy.
7. Stir once again after remove from the pan after a minute or two.
8. Serve hot.

LUNCH

Creamed Spinach (Page - 30)

DINNER

Pork Chops with Caramelized Onion (Page - 56)

DAY 2

BREAKFAST

Chia Pudding (Page - 21)

LUNCH

Lemon Chicken (Serves 3/ 25 min)

Serving: 1
Net carbs: 4g / 0.14oz
Fiber: 4g / 0.14oz
Fat: 9g / 0.32oz
Protein: 49g / 1.73oz
kcal: 307

INGREDIENTS:

- 1 lb Chicken Breast
- 2 tsp Ghee/ Melted Butter
- ¼ Lemon Slices
- 1 tbsp Lemon Juice
- ¼ tsp Kosher Salt
- 1 tbsp Water
- 1 ½ cup Broccoli Florets

INSTRUCTIONS:

1. Heat up ghee/ butter in a large pan. Keep the heat over medium-high.
2. Season chicken breast with kosher salt and add to the pan.
3. Cook on one side for about 10 minutes. Flip the chicken and add lemon slices. Cook for another 10 minutes.
4. Add broccoli, lemon juice and water. Cover with a lid and cook until the internal temperature of the chicken reaches 165 F.
5. Remove from the pan. Serve warm with cauliflower rice.

DINNER

Eggplant Parmesan (Page - 54)

DAY 3

BREAKFAST

Mocha Mousse (Page - 25)

LUNCH

Fried Cauliflower and Cheese Patties (Page - 29)

DINNER

Swedish Meatballs (Serves 6/ 30 min)

Serving: 1
Net carbs: 3.2g / 0.11 oz
Fiber: 2g / 0.07 oz
Fat: 11.25g / 0.39 oz
Protein: 7g / 0.25 oz
kcal: 243

INGREDIENTS:

- 1 lb Ground Pork
- 1 cup Chicken Broth
- 1 lb Ground Chuck
- 1 Egg
- 3/4 cup Heavy Cream
- 1 cup Zucchini (Grated)
- 1/4 tsp Salt
- 1 tsp All-Purpose Seasoning
- 2 tbsp Butter
- 1 tbsp Mustard

INSTRUCTIONS:

1. Add ground pork, ground chuck, grated zucchini, egg, salt and all-purpose seasoning in a mixing bowl. Combine well.
2. Shape the mixture into 18 small balls.

3. Melt the butter in a large skillet.
4. Add the meatballs and cook for 10 minutes until both sides turn brownish.
5. Whisk the chicken broth, heavy cream and mustard in a separate bowl.
6. Pour over the meatballs and let the sauce simmer for 5-10 minutes.
7. Remove from the skillet when the sauce has thickened up. Serve hot.

DAY 4

BREAKFAST

Cream Cheese Pancakes (Serves 3/ 10min)

Serving: 1
Net carbs: 3g / 0.10oz
Fat: 29g / 1.02oz
Protein: 17g / 0.59oz
kcal: 349

INGREDIENTS:

- 2 oz Cream Cheese
- 2 large Eggs
- 1/3 tsp Cinnamon Powder
- 1/3 tsp Baking Powder
- 2-3 drops of liquid Stevia
- 1/2 tsp Vanilla Extract

INSTRUCTIONS:

1. Blend all the ingredients in a food processor until a smooth consistency forms.
2. Pour the batter on a non-stick frying pan.
3. Flip when the sides turn brownish.
4. Serve hot with melted butter and your favourite toppings.

LUNCH

Cobb Salad (Page - 38)

DINNER

Shrimp Alfredo (Page - 64)

DAY 5

BREAKFAST

Strawberry Smoothie (Page - 23)

LUNCH

Fried Salmon with Asparagus (Serves 2/15 min)

Serving: 1
Net carbs: 2g / 0.07oz
Fiber: 2g / 0.07oz
Fat: 52g / 1.83oz
Protein: 28g / 0.99oz
kcal: 591

INGREDIENTS:

- 9 oz Salmon
- 8 oz Asparagus
- 3 oz Butter
- Salt and Pepper (To Taste)

INSTRUCTIONS:

1. Clean the asparagus and trim the edges.
2. Cut the salmon into desired portions.
3. Heat up the butter in a large frying pan.
4. Place the asparagus and cook for 3-4 minutes over medium heat. Add salt and pepper. Slide the asparagus to one corner of the pan.
5. Add more butter if necessary and place the salmon on the pan.
6. Cook for a few minutes on each side until the whole fish is cooked.
7. Remove from the pan and serve with the asparagus and butter from the pan.

DINNER

Chicken & Mushroom Stew (Page - 51)

DAY 6

BREAKFAST

Vegan Porridge (Page - 16)

LUNCH

Bacon & Cheeseburger Soup (Page - 35)

DINNER

Pizza on a Skillet (Serves 1/ 25 min)

Serving: 1
Net carbs: 5g / 0.18oz
Fiber: 1g / 0.03oz
Fat: 50g / 1.76oz
Protein: 33g / 1.16oz
kcal: 606

INGREDIENTS:

- 3 oz shredded Mozzarella Cheese
- 1 oz sliced Pepperoni
- 2 oz Sausage (Cooked and Crumbled)
- 1 oz Bell Peppers (Thinly Sliced)
- ½ tsp Italian Seasoning
- 2 tbsp Tomato Sauce

INSTRUCTIONS:

1. Heat up a 8" non-stick skillet.
2. Add 3/4 of the mozzarella cheese to cover the bottom of the skillet.
3. Once the cheese has melted, add tomato sauce, sausage, bell pepper slices. Add another layer of cheese and top with the pepperoni.
4. Cook for 3-4 minutes in low heat.

5. Add Italian seasoning on top as the cheese on the top starts to meltdown.
6. Turn off the heat and allow it to cool down for 5 minutes or so.
7. Serve warm.

DAY 7

BREAKFAST

Eggs & Mayo (Serves 2/ 8 min)

Serving: 1
Net carbs: 1g / 0.03oz
Fat: 29g / 1.02oz
Protein: 11g / 0.39oz
kcal: 316

INGREDIENTS:

- 4 medium-sized Eggs
- 4 tbsp homemade Mayonnaise
- Pinch of Ground Pepper
- Pinch of Chopped Parsley

INSTRUCTIONS:

1. Boil water in a medium-sized pot.
2. Place the eggs and cook for 8-10 minutes. You will get hard-boiled eggs.
3. Cut the eggs in halves and season with pepper and parsley.
4. Serve with mayonnaise.

LUNCH

Oven-Baked Chicken Parmesan (Page - 39)

DINNER

Thai Spicy Tofu (Page - 66)

DAY 8

BREAKFAST

French Toast from Scratch (Page - 19

LUNCH

Dill Pickles in Bacon Wraps (Serves 4/35 min)

Serving: 4
Net carbs: 2g / 0.7oz
Fat: 7g / 0.25oz
Protein: 5g / 0.17oz
kcal: 80

INGREDIENTS:

- 8 slices of uncooked Bacon
- 4 Dill Pickles
- 2 tbsp homemade Ranch dressing
- Pinch of Kosher Salt
- Pinch of Ground Pepper

INSTRUCTIONS:

1. Slice the bacon into halves. You will get 16 slices of bacon.
2. Cut the dill pickles into quarters. Remove excess moisture with a paper towel.
3. Preheat the oven to 425 F.
4. Place a piece of pickle in the middle of a bacon slice. Wrap it and secure with a toothpick.
5. Grease a baking sheet lined with parchment paper.
6. Bake for 25-30 minutes until the bacon turns crispy.
7. Sprinkle salt and pepper.
8. Serve warm with the Ranch dressing.

DINNER

Buffalo Chicken Soup (Page - 52)

DAY 9

BREAKFAST

Cheesy Breakfast Bowl (Page - 27)

LUNCH

Lunchbox Omelette (Page - 47)

DINNER

Coconut Salmon and Napa Cabbage (Serves 4/ 30 min)

Serving: 1
Net carb: 3g/ 0.10oz
Fiber: 3g / 0.10oz
Fat: 67g / 2.36oz
Protein: 32g / 0.13oz
kcal: 744

INGREDIENTS:

- 1¼ lbs Salmon
- ½ cup Shredded Coconut
- 1¼ lbs Napa Cabbage
- 1 tbsp Olive Oil
- 4 oz. butter
- 1 tsp Turmeric Powder
- ½ tsp Onion Powder
- 1 tsp Kosher Salt
- 4 tbsp Olive Oil (For Frying)
- Pinch of Salt
- Pinch of Pepper
- 2 Lemon Slices

INSTRUCTIONS:

1. Cut the salmon into 1 x 1-inch bite-size pieces. Drizzle with 1 tbsp olive oil.
2. Take a mixing bowl and combine the shredded coconut, salt, turmeric powder and onion powder.
3. Put the salmon pieces in the mixture and coat well.
4. Fry the salmon on medium-high heat until they turn golden brown.
5. Chop the cabbage into long strips and fry them with butter. Remove from pan when they are caramelized. Add a seasoning of salt and pepper.
6. Serve with the salmon cubes, juice from the pan and fresh lemon slices.

DAY 10

BREAKFAST

Butter Coffee (Serves 1/ 5min)

Serving: 1
Fat: 38g / 1.27oz
Protein: 1g / 0.03 oz
kcal: 334

INGREDIENTS:

- 1 cup hot coffee (Freshly Brewed)
- 1 tbsp Coconut Oil
- 2 tbsp unsalted butter
- 2/3 drops of liquid Stevia

INSTRUCTIONS:

1. Melt the butter in the microwave.
2. Combine with the coconut oil and stevia.
3. Pour the hot coffee and blend everything together.
4. Sip into the delicious and healthy drink.

LUNCH

Cheesy Lettuce Wraps (Page - 36)

DINNER

Oven-baked Meatloaf (Page - 57)

DAY 11

BREAKFAST

Sausage Casserole (Page - 15)

LUNCH

Goat Cheese Salad Bowl (Serves 2/15 min)

>Serving: 1
>Net carbs: 3g / 1.5oz
>Fiber: 2g / 0.07oz
>Fat: 73g / 0.80oz
>Protein: 37g / 1.5oz
>kcal: 824

INGREDIENTS:

- 10 oz Goat Cheese
- 3 oz. Baby Spinach
- ¼ cup Pumpkin Seeds
- 1 tbsp Balsamic Vinegar
- 2 oz unsalted butter

INSTRUCTIONS:

1. Pre-heat oven to 400°F.
2. Grease a baking dish with non-stick cooking spray. Place slices of goat cheese and bake for 10 minutes.
3. While the cheese is being cooked in the oven, toast the pumpkin seeds in a frying pan for 2-3 minutes.
4. Decrease the heat to low and add butter. Let the mixture simmer until they turn golden brown.

5. Pour in the balsamic vinegar. Boil for a few minutes and remove from the pan.
6. Lay the baby spinach on a serving bowl. Add cheese and roasted seeds. Eat while it's warm.

DINNER

Asian-style Stir-Fried Veggies (Page - 67)

DAY 12

BREAKFAST

Crunchy Energy Bars (Page - 24)

LUNCH

Zucchini Bolognese (Page - 42)

DINNER

Chicken Chili (Serves 6/ 30 min)

Serving: 1
Net carbs: 7g / 0.25oz
Fiber: 1g / 0.03oz
Fat: 11g / 0.39oz
Protein: 18g / 0.63oz
kcal: 201

INGREDIENTS:

- 4 Chicken Breasts (Shredded)
- 2 cups Chicken Broth
- 1 tbsp Butter
- 10 oz Tomatoes (Diced)
- ½ Onion (Chopped)
- 2 oz Tomato Puree
- 1 tbsp Cumin Powder
- 1 tbsp Chili Powder
- 1/2 tbsp Garlic Powder
- 1 Jalapeno Pepper (Thinly Sliced)
- 4 oz Cream cheese
- Salt and pepper to taste

INSTRUCTIONS:

1. Melt butter in a large stockpot. Keep the heat over medium-high. Sautee the onion until it turns translucent.
2. Add the shredded chicken, diced tomatoes, tomato paste, cum-

in powder, chili powder, garlic powder and sliced jalapeno.

3. Pour the chicken broth. Stir everything and bring it to a boil.
4. Decrease the heat to low and cover with a lid. Let it simmer for 10 minutes.
5. Chop the cream cheese into small cubes.
6. Add the cream cheese to the mixture.
7. Turn up the heat to medium-high. Stir to combine the cheese with the mixture.
8. Remove from the pan when the cheese is blended and serve hot.

DAY 13

BREAKFAST

Chocolate Milkshake (Serves 1/ 5min)

Serving: 1
Net carbs: 10.75g / 0.38oz
Fiber: 5.5g / 0.19oz
Fat: 31g / 1.09oz
Protein: 3g / 0.10oz
kcal: 303

INGREDIENTS:

- ½ cup Coconut Milk
- 1/2 medium-sized Avocado
- 1-2 tbsp Cocoa Powder
- 1/2 tsp Vanilla Extract
- Pinch of Salt
- Ice Cubes
- Sweetener of choice

INSTRUCTIONS:

1. Blend all the ingredients in a blender till you get a smooth consistency.
2. Add more sweetener if needed.
3. Drink up!

LUNCH

Indian Style Chicken Curry (Page - 31)

DINNER

Mashed Cauliflower (Page - 50)

DAY 14

BREAKFAST

Ham & Cheese Pockets (Page - 18)

LUNCH

Deli Lunch Box (Serves 1/15 min)

Serving: 1
Net carbs: 16g / 0.56oz
Fat: 25g / 0.88oz
Protein: 23g / 0.81oz
kcal: 382.2

INGREDIENTS:

- 2 oz Turkey Breast (Thinly Sliced)
- 1 hard-boiled Egg (Sliced half)
- 1/4 cup Cherry Tomatoes (Sliced Half)
- 1 oz Cheddar Cheese (Cubed)
- 2 tbsp roasted Almonds
- 4 Pita Bites Crackers

INSTRUCTIONS:

1. Place all the ingredients in a lunch box.
2. Make sure the ingredients are not all scattered over each other.

DINNER

Salisbury Steak in Slow Cooker (Page - 60)

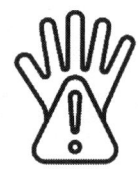

Disclaimer

The opinions and ideas of the author contained in this publication are designed to educate the reader in an informative and helpful manner. While we accept that the instructions will not suit every reader, it is only to be expected that the recipes might not gel with everyone. Use the book responsibly and at your own risk. This work with all its contents, does not guarantee correctness, completion, quality or correctness of the provided information. Always check with your medical practitioner should you be unsure whether to follow a low carb eating plan. Misinformation or misprints cannot be completely eliminated. Human error is real!

Design: JustCreate

Picture: Timolina / www.shutterstock.com

[Handwritten notes:]

Pancake
- almond flour
- cream cheese
- sweetener
- eggs
- cinnamon

Printed in Great Britain
by Amazon